KETO FOR WOMEN

OVER 50

The Simplified Guide to A Ketogenic

Diet Lifestyle For Women Over 50

Burn Fat Forever, Reverse Diabetes &

Lower Your Triglycerides Effectively

With A Gentler Approach

Katie Simmons

Text   Copyright

Legal & Disclaimer

disclaimer applies to any loss, damages or injury caused by the use and application, whether directly or indirectly, of any advice or information presented, whether for breach of contract, tort, negligence, personal injury, criminal intent, or under any other cause of action.

You agree to accept all risks of using the information presented inside this book.

You agree that by continuing to read this book, where appropriate and/or necessary, you shall consult a professional (including but not limited to your doctor, attorney, or financial advisor or such other advisor as needed) before using any of the suggested remedies, techniques, or information in this book.

Introduction

Keto diet has embraced a lot of appreciation and praise due to its weight loss benefits. This high fat and low carb diet has proven to be extremely healthy overall. It actually makes your body burn fat, like a machine which is why; public figures are also highly appreciative of it. But the question is how does ketosis boost weight loss? Here is a detailed insight to the process of ketosis and weight loss.

Ketosis is considered abnormal by some people. Despite the fact that it has been approved by a lot of nutritionists and doctors; a lot of people still disapprove of it. The misconceptions are all due to the myths that have been spread around about the ketogenic diet.

Ketogenic diet is a normal diet plan and the process of ketosis is a normal, metabolic function. The rule is to lower the blood sugar levels so that the body accesses the stored, extra fat to produce energy.

Once your body does not have glucose, it is automatically going to rely on the stored fat. Also, it is important to understand that carbs create glucose and once you start taking a low carb diet, you will be able to lower the glucose levels as well. Thus, your body is going to create the fuel through fats, instead of carbs, that is glucose.

The process of creating fuel through fat is known as ketosis and once your body enters this state, it becomes extremely efficient in burning the unwanted fat. Also, as glucose levels are low during ketogenic diet, your body attains a lot of other health benefits as well.

This is how your body burns fat rapidly during ketosis, providing you with intense and amazing weight loss outcomes. Ketogenic diet is not just helpful for weight loss but also aids in boosting your overall health in positive ways. Unlike all the other diet plans, which focus on cutting down your caloric intake, keto emphasis on putting your body in a natural metabolic state, that is ketosis. The only factor that makes this diet plan doubtful is that this nature of metabolism is not talked about a lot. With your body producing ketones regularly, your body will burn the stored fat swiftly which will result in great weight loss.

Now, the query arises; how does ketosis affect the human body?

The truth is that ketogenic diet is healthy for almost everyone. However, one needs to accept that this diet plan is totally different from the ones that we usually try. Thus, your body is definitely going to react a little to the new process. The side effects are termed as "keto flu" during which, one might experience extreme hunger, low energy levels, bad sleeping pattern and a little nauseous as well.

However, this phase does not last longer than 2-3 days. This is the time required by the human body to enter the phase of ketosis. Once you have entered it, you are hardly going to have any adverse side effects.

Moreover, you need to start limiting your caloric and carb intake gradually. The most common mistake that keto dieters make is that they tend to start cutting off everything from their diet, all at once. This is where the issue arises. The human body will react extremely negative when you will restrict everything right away. You need to start gradually. Read this guide for more on how to approach keto diet after 50.

Chapter 1 How Keto Diet Works

What Is Ketogenic Diet?

You all know that our body needs energy for its functioning and the energy sources come from carbohydrates, proteins, and fats. Owing to years of conditioning that a low-fat carbohydrate-rich diet is essential for good health, we have become used to depending on glucose (from carbohydrates) to get most of the energy that our body needs. Only when the amount of glucose available for energy generation decreases, does our body begin to break down fat for drawing energy to power our cells and organs. This is the express purpose of a ketogenic diet.

The primary aim of a ketogenic diet (called simply as keto diet) is to convert your body into a fat-burning machine. Such a diet is loaded with benefits and is highly recommended by nutritional experts for the following end results:

•Natural appetite control

•Increased mental clarity

•Lowered levels of inflammation in the body system

•Improved stability in blood sugar levels

•Elimination or lower risk of heartburn

• Using natural stored body fat as the fuel source

•Weight loss

The effects listed are just some of the numerous effects that take place when a person embarks on a ketogenic diet and makes it a point to stick to it. A ketogenic diet consists of meals with low carbohydrates, moderate proteins, and high-fat content. The mechanism works like this: when we drastically reduce the intake of carbohydrates, our body is compelled to convert fat for releasing energy. This process of converting fats instead of carbohydrates to release energy is called ketosis.

How Does The Ketogenic Diet Work?

The time has come for you to get the answer to the question that has been lingering in your mind from the time you heard about the keto diet; 'how does a keto diet work?'

Here is how.

The power behind the Ketogenic diet's ability to help you lose weight and have better health comes from one simple action that the diet initiates in your body once you start following it. This simple action is how the keto diet changes your metabolism from burning carbohydrates for energy to burning fats for energy.

What does that have to do with weight loss and better health?

Let me break it down for you.

•   Burning carbohydrate for energy

Most of the food we eat follow the food pyramid recommended by the USDA some few decades ago. The pyramid puts carbohydrates at the bottom of the pyramid and fats at the top of the pyramid, which essentially means that carbohydrates form the bulk of the foods we eat, as shown below:

What many of us don't know is that when you consume a diet that is high in carbohydrate, two things normally happen.

•   One, your body takes the just consumed carbohydrates and converts it into glucose which is the easiest molecule that your body can convert to use as energy (glucose is your body's primary source of energy, as it gets chosen over any other energy source in your body).

•   Secondly, your body produces insulin for the sole purpose of it moving the glucose from your bloodstream into your cells where it can be used as energy.

There is more that goes unnoticed though:

Since your body gets its energy from glucose (which is mostly in huge amounts owing to the fact that we eat lots of high carb food 3-6 times a day), it doesn't need any other source of energy. In fact, many are the times when glucose is in excess, something that prompts the body to convert dietary glucose into glycogen to be stored in the liver and muscle cells. But since glycogen stores tend to be quite limited, the excess glucose is converted into fatty acids and glycerol, which is stored in fat stores around the body in the form of triglycerides. What this simple explanation means is that with a high carb diet, your body is essentially in what we refer to as a fat-storing mode. It stores this excess fat so that it can use it when starved from its primary source of energy; glucose. Unfortunately, since we don't give ourselves enough breaks from food, we end up being in this constant fat-storing mode that ultimately causes weight gain.

•   Burning fats for energy

As you now know, the Ketogenic diet is a low carb, high fat, and moderate protein diet. So when you start following a Ketogenic diet, what typically happens is, your intake of carbohydrate is kept at a low. In other words, it inverts the USDA food pyramid I mentioned earlier, something that literally 'inverts/reverses' the effects of a high carb diet.

How exactly does it do that?

Well, when you limit your carb intake greatly, you starve the body of its primary source of energy, something that initiates the process that the body has always been preparing for through its energy storage processes. More specifically, the body starts by metabolizing glycogen with the help of glucagon hormone (the process takes place in the liver). And with support from the human growth hormone, cortisol, and catecholamines (norepinephrine to be more specific), the body starts releasing fatty acids for use as energy in different body parts. But since fatty acids cannot be used by every cell in the body, the body is also forced to transport some of the fatty acids to the liver where they are broken down in a series of metabolic processes known as ketosis to produce 3 ketone bodies. Therefore, Ketosis is a natural process that your body activates when your energy intake is low for the purpose of helping you to survive. The three ketones that are formed when fatty acids are converted are:

• Acetone.

• Beta-hydroxybutyric acid (BHB)

• Acetoacetate (AcAc)

Many of your body cells (including the brain cells) can use BHB for energy, as it is water-soluble, something that makes it very much like glucose in that it can cross the-blood brain barrier. The more ketones the body cells use for energy, the more fat you are burning and ultimately, the more weight you stand to gain. Keep in mind that you are also taking lots of dietary fats. The reason for taking lots of dietary fats is to fill you up fast, make you to stay full for longer and accustom the body cells to using fatty acids and ketones for energy so that when the deficit created by dietary fats kicks in (because you are unlikely to eat so much fats to the point of meeting your body's energy requirements- unless you are gluttonous), you begin burning stored body fat immediately, as opposed to starting with glycogen. Moderate intake of protein also helps you to get filled fast and to stay full for longer. Keeping your protein intake moderate is therefore vital, as any excess may end up causing you to get out of ketosis, as excess protein may be metabolized to glucose in a process known as gluconeogenesis. This essentially means a Ketogenic diet makes your body a fat-burning machine, as it relies primarily on fats (both dietary and stored body fat – though you want to get your body to burn as much of the stored boy fat as possible).

Ketosis helps you get rid of excessive fats in your body, which not only reduce your weight in an immense way but also betters your health by protecting you from various diseases as you will see later on.

To attain ketosis, you know that your intake of fats should be high, intake of carbs low and intake of proteins moderate. But what exactly does high, low and moderate translate to in calorie terms? In simpler terms, in what ratios should you take carbs, fats, and proteins? This gives rise to several types/approaches/schools of thought regarding the ratios:

The History of the Ketogenic Diet

The ketogenic diet traces its roots to the treatment of epilepsy. Surprisingly this goes all the way back to 500 BC, when ancient Greeks observed that fasting or eating a ketogenic diet helped reduce epileptic seizures. In modern times, the ketogenic diet was reintroduced in the practice of medicine to treat children with epilepsy. In 1921, a scientist named Rollin Woodyatt discovered that the liver made ketone bodies during starvation or when the patient was following a high fat, low carbohydrate diet.

Research into the keto diet stalled until the 1960s, when scientists discovered that a certain class of fats called medium chain triglycerides or MCTs were readily transported to the liver and made into ketone bodies, faster than normal fats (coconut oil is an example). It was also found that the body could go into a state of ketosis eating more protein when large amounts of MCTs were consumed.

In the early 1970s, a cardiologist named Robert Atkins proposed his own version of a ketogenic diet called the Atkins diet, which has been immensely popular. The Atkins diet has more relaxed standards that keto, allowing adherents to follow very strict carbohydrate consumption for the first two weeks during an "induction phase." After this, the number of carbohydrates consumed can be slightly increased.

From there, research on ketogenic diets stalled again. However, in the past fifteen years, there has been an explosion of interest in the diet.

Chapter 2 Keto Diet Types

The ketogenic diet seems fairly simple, but there is no one way to do it. To have the most favorable outcomes with a diet, it is important that it fits well with you and your lifestyle. That's why there are a few different options with keto.

Each has a small variation on carbohydrate versus fat intake to meet your needs and your health goals. What kind of diet you follow will also be determined by your desire to eat meat or to be vegetarian. When you choose which one suits you best, you must ensure that you have clear goals in mind. You may have to experiment a bit to find what works for you.

The standard ketogenic diet (SKD)

The standard keto diet is the most popular version. With SKD, the number of net carbohydrates is kept between 25-50 g, but this is not set in stone. It focuses on keeping very low, sufficient amounts of protein and lots of fat.

The targeted ketogenic diet (TKD)

This version is more aimed at people who are very athletic and feel the need to eat 25-50 g of carbohydrates within 30 minutes before they start exercising to achieve maximum performance. The amount of carbohydrates you 'need' is still being discussed fiercely, so we encourage experiments.

The cyclic ketogenic diet (CKD)

If you have never tried keto, the cyclic ketogenic approach can relieve some of the pressure. It means that periods of carbohydrate-restricted eating are alternated with periods of more carbohydrates (no junk food party!). This version is great to gain insight into when you feel in and out of ketosis. Be careful because you cannot get in and out every day; it is more keto for a few weeks and then no keto for a few days.

Chapter 3 Why For Over 50

The transition or menopause happens when a woman has had no menstruation for longer than a year. Usually, the phenomenon happens in women over the age of 50. It is an indication that the fertile years in the life of a woman have arrived at an end. The menstrual cycle is directed by a series of processes in the mind, ovaries, and womb. These provide a hormone balance in which the following hormones are included:

Estrogen

FSH (follicle stimulating hormone)

LH (luteinizing hormone)

Progesterone

The menopause modifies this hormonal balance. The creation of progesterone and estrogen is reduced, while the creation of FSH and LH rises. This modification triggers a large number of physical changes. Certainly, estrogen and progesterone also impact other body organs and cells in the body. Lots of people recognize these menopause signs and symptoms:

Mood swings

Hot flashes

Sweating nightly

Decrease of libido

Insomnia

Undesirable urine loss

Vaginal drought

This is a small list of various other symptoms that are triggered by the effects on the metabolic process:

Delayed metabolism

Glucose intolerance

Insulin resistance

Weight gain

Higher cholesterol

There's a whole lot that the ketogenic diet does to help you reach a healthy and balanced weight and stay there: restore insulin levels of sensitivity, build and maintain muscle mass, and lower inflammation. A woman who consumes way too many carbohydrates can jump start menopause signs. Let's have a look at how a ketogenic diet can aid with the signs and symptoms of this menopause.

Way # 1 - Controlling Insulin Levels

By going on a ketogenic diet, women with PCOS (polycystic-over-the-air disorder) can help regulate their hormones. A research study on the effect of low-glycemic diets has shown this impact. PCOS triggers insulin sensitivity concerns, which can be helped by the insulin-reducing properties of low-glycemic carbohydrates.

Way # 2 - You'll have much more energy

Our bodies will experience widely known energy dips if we fuel them with mainly sugar and carbohydrates. Especially if you take in quick and refined sugars (think about carrot cake, cupcakes, crackers, bread, candy, etc.). Changes in blood glucose can be stopped by receiving a steady amount of sugar. High blood glucose makes the body send insulin to the pancreas, which then begins to take care of the way in which muscular tissue and fat cells absorb sugar.

The reaction to the consumption of carbs is a powerful release of insulin to make sure that body can properly manage the transport of the new sugar. With blood sugar levels down, the body will signal that it requires more sugar. This means that you'll experience many energy lows and highs in one day. This produces a reduced energy level.

Way # 3 - Fat burning

Menopause can trigger the metabolic process to change and reduce. One of the most common complaints of the menopause is an increase in body weight and abdominal fat. A lower level of estrogen typically causes weight gain. A diet with little or no carbohydrates is very efficient for decreasing body fat. Additionally, ketosis reduces appetite by controlling the production of the 'cravings hormonal agent' called ghrelin. You are generally less hungry while in ketosis.

Way # 4 - Hot flashes will be reduced

Nobody totally understands hot flashes and why they take place. Hormonal changes that impact the hypothalamus, most likely have something to do with this. The hypothalamus manages the body's temperature level. Changes in hormonal agents can also disrupt this thermostat. This ends up being more sensitive to modifications in body temperature levels.

Ketones, the production of which is stimulated throughout a ketogenic diet, create a very potent source of energy for the mind. Scientists have demonstrated that ketones act to help the hypothalamus. The body will have the ability to manage its own temperature level better. The presence of ketones works to make your body's thermostat better.

Way # 5 - Excellent night's rest

Thanks to a much more steady blood sugar level, you will improve rest while on a ketogenic diet. With even more balanced hormones and much less warm flashes, you will sleep better as well. Reduced stress and an enhanced well-being are 2 of the benefits of better sleep.

Chapter 4 Differences Between Old And Young Women During A Keto Diet

The ketogenic diet provides the body with premium fuel in the form of fats that make you fitter and younger with the energy of a twenty-year-old and the best part, it lasts longer than carb fuel.

By following the ketogenic diet, you can lose all the unwanted weight without ever stepping foot in a gym, without any meal portion control or counting calories. The ketogenic diet has proven to work for people with all types of background and health issues like having blood sugar issues, obesity, post-pregnancy, people having food addictions, those who are suffering from emotional eating, etc. Before going into more details about keto diet, specifically for seniors over 50, let's dive into its history.

The ketogenic diet is nothing new; it has been in existence for over ninety years. The Keto diet was designed by Dr. Russell Wilder in 1924 as a treatment for his epileptic patients. He found out that fasting which led body into ketosis was proving fruitful to control the epileptic seizures in their patient, but fasting wasn't a permanent solution. Hence, they came up with a high-fat and low-carb diet for the patients that worked equally and that too effectively as a cure for epilepsy when no medicine could help. With more research on this diet, the keto diet began being successfully used to treat a variety of other medical conditions, especially obesity. Other benefits apart from epilepsy and losing a few pounds of weights are:

- Alzheimer's disease

- Parkinson's disease

- Multiple Sclerosis

- Healing traumatic brain injuries

- Improve cardiovascular health

- Prevent heart attack and stroke

- Reduce and maintain healthy blood sugar levels

- Fight various kinds of cancer

- Treat Autism

- Decrease acne

- Decrease risk factors for polycystic ovary syndrome and respiratory disease

Our body functions and performs its processes differently at a senior age compared to when it is 20 or 30 years old because, at this age, the metabolism is too slow to burn off any extra calories or fats. This is, unfortunately, a sad reality, but it doesn't mean that a person over 50 cannot implement a ketogenic lifestyle. Off course you can, The ketogenic diet is a varied diet, and you just have to do few changes in it and adjust to it in a precise way.

Ketogenic diet supports very low or zero-carbs in the diet. And this is not good in the initial days when the body is in the process of transitioning to a Keto diet. We have always been eating so many carbs that handling this sudden change in the food for our body gets challenging and you end up suffering from Keto flu. And with more age, your body has a more difficult time in adjusting and overcoming the side effects for adapting to keto diet. The younger generation has a robust support system, but over the age of 50, the side effect hits you harder and you take more time to recover. You may experience fatigue, headache, nausea, dizziness, lack of motivation and difficulty in focusing. These symptoms are enough to discourage anyone who is finally ready to take charge of their health and body once again, and this stops you from getting the healthy changes you deserve. But don't feel low and worried. Even at this age, the keto diet will work fine for you, and you can still utilize all the incredible benefits of the Ketogenic diet.

Do you know that eating more fats during a ketogenic diet might actually prevent you from having a heart stroke. Why? There is a general misconception that fats clog arteries, but that is not the case with the ketogenic diet because you are actually burning fats on the keto diet and as a result, lose weight.

Here are some simple rules that always work for adhering to the ketogenic diet without any difficulty and headache.

Rule # 1: No Carbs

The main aim of the ketogenic diet is to have carbs as low as possible. You cannot consume foods that are high in carbs, except for veggies. In the initial days of your ketogenic diet, you can stick to 5 to 10 percent of carbs in your meals, about 20 grams, not more than that or else your body will take a lot of time to get into ketosis. And with time, you have to decrease the carbs and go to zero level.

Rule # 2: Have a fatty meal

Most of the keto-ers fail to realize that they should load their body with as many fats as possible during the first meal of the day – breakfast. For example, you can have a quick fatty breakfast in the form of keto coffee mixed with MCT oil or high-fat butter. Or, you can have your regular breakfast consisting of eggs, bacon, and avocado. Your goal should be to get one-third portion of fat for the day from breakfast. For the rest of day, get most of the fat from fatty meats, cheeses, nuts, avocado oil, one or two cups of salad greens and coconut milk.

Rule # 3: Don't go high in protein

The ketogenic diet allows just enough protein that is essential to maintain growth; it's not a high-protein diet. In the beginning you will take time to know the right amount of protein you should consume. However, you can start with having grass-fed and fatty meat of about a fist, twice a day. This rule of getting protein into your body is not perfect, but it is a simple starting point until you figure out how you much protein you need. The best fatty meats are beef, skin-on chicken thighs, pork, salmon, lamb, wild games and eggs. Remember that you cannot have too much meat on the keto diet. Start with taking two fists amount of meat regularly and then cut back to one and a half fist.

Rule # 4: Don't restrict calories

The significant benefit of the keto diet is its inadvertent calorie restriction. If you are not convinced of this, then try this rule for three weeks. For three weeks, don't do a calorie count of your meals and don't weight and measure. Eat until you are satisfied and not hungry anymore; don't eat until you are bursting. After three weeks, check your weight and if it declines then keep following this rule.

Follow these four rules, and you should have no problem in getting your body into ketosis and staying in this state. The three to four weeks might be a little rough, but if you are stick with keto as closely as possible, you will find that the keto diet is easy to live on and its amazing wonders. Once you are there and the fat-burning is built, you are good to go.

Chapter 5 How To Start After 50

Adaptation of ketosis can be tough and you will need time to adjust to the changes. It is normal and everyone faces troubles in adapting to any new dietary plan. However, here are some steps to help you in transiting into ketogenic diet plan perfectly. Just remember that it does require time and you will have to give yourself a little space to adjust to the restrictions. It won't happen overnight to don't be disheartened and stay motivated!

• Gain Knowledge:

The most basic mistake that a lot of keto dieters make is that they don't gain enough knowledge, before starting the diet itself. Therefore, the most important step is to gain knowledge and learn the small differences that make a huge difference. Understand what keto friendly foods are what foods are not meant for ketosis at all. For example, a lot of apple does not eat an apple because it has a lot of carbs. However, if you have a medium or a small sized apple, then you are good to have it. As long as it remains within your carb limit, it is keto friendly. You can also eat an apple a day (depending on the size) but you need to remember the essence of ketosis and take your carbs from energetic sources like protein and healthy fats. Once you are able to understand the difference between non-keto and keto-friendly foods; you will notice that ketosis is not that tough after all.

- Calculation is Important:

The best way to transit in ketosis is to keep a track of your carbs. This might seem annoying at first, but gradually, you will see how helpful it is and you will eventually understand the importance of calculating the net carbs per day. It is extremely crucial and usually people overlook this issue quite easily. However, if you want to settle into ketosis perfectly; it is best that you keep a track of your net carbs.

- Set an Environment:

Most of the people who struggle at ketosis are the ones who don't set their environment according to it. Stocking up your fridge is the basic step towards settling your environment. You certainly cannot expect your surroundings to be filled with ice cream, candies, chocolates and nuts and hope to settle for a huge dietary lifestyle change, can you? It is somewhat impossible. Thus, the best way to transit into ketosis, is to set your atmosphere accordingly. Clean your pantry, make a list of healthy, low carb foods and go to the grocery store to stock up on them. Bring a limitation to the variety of food that is accessible at your home and plan your meals ahead. Put a meal plan in front of your desk every week, so that you always have an eye on it.

- Mindful Eating:

Mindful eating is a very important step towards transition into ketosis. Your caloric intake has a huge impact on your weight loss. The more calories you take, the harder it gets to lose the stubborn, stored fat. A keto calculator can be extremely helpful in this matter though. You can calculate your caloric intake on the go and limit your food intake accordingly. Also, before you pick something to eat, you can instantly calculate the calories you will be take in. This is known as mindful eating; knowing what you are eating and how is it going to affect you.

Ketosis is all about gaining knowledge and getting into the habit of mindful eating. Once you have the knowledge about what you are eating and how much does it has to offer to you; you are gradually going to see major changes taking place in your overall diet routine. You will also find yourself adjusting to ketosis much easier.

Chapter 6   Differences   Between   Old   And Young Women During A Keto Diet

As your body ages, your diet should change. The diets that work well for people in their 20's may not yield the same result for those in their 30's or 50's. 50 is that stage of life when you should start to slow down and take things easy, lest you want to run the risk of getting into accidents.

Sadly, no one is spared from this problem. Both men and women have this problem, even if they have been leading active lifestyles, although women have it a lot worse than men.

It does not happen instantly when you hit the magic number, either. Your body has been starting to slow down since you hit 30. You may notice certain anomalies like you can no longer party until 6 in the morning. But what is the science behind this?

Simply put, as we age, our lean muscle mass goes down, which slows our metabolism down. That, along with our not-as-active lifestyle when we get older, means that our body does not get to burn as many calories as it used to. All this contributes to weight gain. In the past, we could just cut out a snack and magically lose weight. That just will not cut it anymore when we are over 50.

Women have to undergo hormonal changes. They have to deal with menopause, which causes a lack of estrogen in their body. This leads to a shift of fat to the abdomen, increasing their risk of heart disease, type 2 diabetes, and stroke.

There is a misconception that men have it easier compared to women when it comes to weight loss. This is not true. At around 50, men can lose up to 10 pounds of muscle and the figure will only go up as the years go on. Bones and joints may start to develop pain because of the loss of muscular support, which prompt many to ditch the active lifestyle altogether and take it easy (and gain more weight). Of course, men lose muscle mass and consume more calories compared to women, but the figures change at the magic number. They also experience similar hormonal changes to women's menopause. While women over 50 suffer from the steep decline of estrogen, men's testosterone level dips at that age, which leads to more reduction in metabolism rate.

Other than that, there are a few other factors that play a role in your metabolism rate:

•   Sleep: Sleep helps regulate your hormones and prevent food cravings. People in their fifties should consider going to sleep early to get enough sleep.

•   Heredity: No two people have the same metabolism. Some are blessed and can shed pounds just by weaning off some snacks whereas others get fatter just by looking at a donut. But that does not mean you cannot lose weight. It just takes time and consistency.

• Medication: Certain medications such as anti-depressants, steroids, diabetes and anti-seizure help your body retain fluid, lower metabolism, and make you feel hungrier. These are not side effects because those medications are intended to provide your body with the energy it needs to fight off disease and remain strong. However, if you are looking to lose weight and are on those medications, then consider consulting your doctor and explore alternatives. Don't stop taking your medications outright.

However, just because your age is high does not mean that your weight has to be. Similar to the lifestyle changes from your 20's to your 30's and 40's, all you need is some changes to better suit your 50-year-old body.

Chapter 7 What To Eat And Drink – What Not

What foods are keto?

Foods that fit into the ketogenic diet are non-starchy veggies and low-carb high-fat foods. It also includes various protein sources. Below is a rough list of some of the most nutritious ketogenic foods, which can be fit into a meal plan.

Healthy ketogenic fats

- Avocado

- Seeds

- Olives

- Cacao

- Plant-based oils

- Nuts and nut butter

- Veggies and low-carb fruit

- All kinds of fresh herbs

- Strawberries and melons

- Nonstarchy veggies like broccoli, cauliflower, radishes, greens, zucchini, eggplant, tomato, green beans, cucumber, mushrooms, celery, bok choy, cabbage, artichoke, onions, beets and carrots.

Keto proteins

- Fatty fish like mackerel, salmon and herring

- Chicken with the skin on

- Pork, lamb, beef, bison and goat

- Shellfish

- Organ meats

- Cheese, cottage cheese and unsweetened yogurt

Keto sweeteners

- Stevia

- Monk fruit

- Erythritol

- Other artificial sweeteners

Which foods are not keto?

A ketogenic meal plan is all about eating enough macros, and this means that you can fit in just about any type of foods in this plan except for high carb foods. There are several sources of carbs, which will push your daily limits within a single serving. Below is a list of foods that need to be avoided while on keto.

High Carb foods

- Milk

- Desserts

- Corn

- Potatoes

- Lentils, beans and legume

- Pasta, bread and all grains

- Soda and juice

- Dried fruit and most fruit

- Fried foods and breaded foods

- Sugars: honey, agave, maple, table sugar, etc.

Keto beverages

- Coffee and tea, unsweetened

- Water

- Club soda/sparkling water

- Artificially sweetened beverages

- Green vegetable juices and wheatgrass

- Flavored water with no added sugar

Low carb alcohol

- Light beers

- Wine and champagne

- Bourbon and scotch

- Gin, rum and vodka

Chapter 8 Most Common Mistakes And How To Fix Them

Do you feel like you are giving your all to the keto diet but you still aren't seeing the results you want? You are measuring ketones, working out, and counting your macros, but you still aren't losing the weight you want. Here are the most common mistakes that most people make when beginning the keto diet.

1.   Too Many Snacks

There are many snacks you can enjoy while following the keto diet, like nuts, avocado, seeds, and cheese. But, snacking can be an easy way to get too many calories into the diet while giving your body an easy fuel source besides stored fat. Snacks need to be only used if you frequently hunger between meals. If you aren't extremely hungry, let your body turn to your stored fat for its fuel between meals instead of dietary fat.

2.   Not Consuming Enough Fat

The ketogenic diet isn't all about low carbs. It's also about high fats. You need to be getting about 75 percent of your calories from healthy fats, five percent from carbs, and 20 percent from protein. Fat makes you feel fuller longer, so if you eat the correct amount, you will minimize your carb cravings, and this will help you stay in ketosis. This will help your body burn fat faster.

3.   Consuming Excessive Calories

You may hear people say you can eat what you want on the keto diet as long as it is high in fat. Even though we want that to be true, it is very misleading. Healthy fats need to make up the biggest part of your diet. If you eat more calories than what you are burning, you will gain weight, no matter what you eat because these excess calories get stored as fat. An average adult only needs about 2,000 calories each day, but this will vary based on many factors like activity level, height, and gender.

4.   Consuming a lot of Dairies

For many people, dairy can cause inflammation and keeps them from losing weight. Dairy is a combo food meaning it has carbs, protein, and fats. If you eat a lot of cheese as a snack for the fat content, you are also getting a dose of carbs and protein with that fat. Many people can tolerate dairy, but moderation is the key. Stick with no more than one to two ounces of cheese or cream at each meal. Remember to factor in the protein content.

5.   Consuming a lot of Protein

The biggest mistake that most people make when just beginning the keto diet is consuming too much protein. Excess protein gets converted into glucose in the body called gluconeogenesis. This is a natural process where the body converts the energy from fats and proteins into glucose when glucose isn't available. When following a ketogenic diet, gluconeogenesis happens at different rates to keep body function. Our bodies don't need a lot of carbs, but we do need glucose. You can eat absolute zero carbs, and through gluconeogenesis, your body will convert other substances into glucose to be used as fuel. This is why carbs only make up five percent of your macros. Some parts of our bodies need carbs to survive, like kidney, medulla, and red blood cells. With gluconeogenesis, our bodies make and stores extra glucose as glycogen just in case supplies become too low.

In a normal diet, when carbs are always available, gluconeogenesis happens slowly because the need for glucose is extremely low. Our body runs on glucose and will store excess protein and carbs as fat.

It does take time for our bodies to switch from using glucose to burning fats. Once you are in ketosis, your body will use fat as the main fuel source and will start to store excess protein as glycogen.

6.   Not Getting Enough Water

Water is crucial for your body. Water is needed for all your body does, and this includes burning fat. If you don't drink enough water, it can cause your metabolism to slow down, and this can halt your weight loss. Drinking 64 ounces or one-half gallon every day will help your body burn fat, flush out toxins, and circulate nutrients. When you are just beginning the keto diet, you might need to drink more water since your body will begin to get rid of body fat by flushing it out through urine.

7.   Consuming Too Many Sweets

Some people might indulge in keto brownies and keto cookies that are full of sugar substitute just because their net carb content is low, but you have to remember that you are still eating calories. Eating sweets might increase your carb cravings. Keto sweets are great on occasion; they don't need to be a staple in the diet.

8.   Not Getting Enough Sleep

Getting plenty of sleep is needed in order to lose weight effectively. Without the right amount of sleep, your body will feel stressed, and this could result in your metabolism slowing down. It might cause it to store fat instead of burning fat. When you feel tired, you are more tempted to drink more lattes for energy, eat a snack to give you an extra boost, or order takeout rather than cooking a healthy meal. Try to get between seven and nine hours of sleep each night. Understand that your body uses that time to burn fat without you even lifting a finger.

9.   Low on Electrolytes

Most people will experience the keto flu when you begin this diet. This happens for two reasons when your body changes from burning carbs to burning fat, your brain might not have enough energy, and this, in turn, can cause grogginess, headaches, and nausea. You could be dehydrated, and your electrolytes might be low since the keto diet causes you to urinate often.

Getting the keto flu is a great sign that you are heading in the right direction. You can lessen these symptoms by drinking more water or taking supplements that will balance your electrolytes.

10.   Consuming Hidden Carbs

Many foods look like they are low carb, but they aren't. You can find carbs in salad dressings, sauces, and condiments. Be sure to check nutrition labels before you try new foods to make sure it doesn't have any hidden sugar or carbs. It just takes a few seconds to skim the label, and it might be the difference between whether or not you'll lose weight.

If you have successfully ruled out all of the above, but you still aren't losing weight, you might need to talk with your doctor to make sure you don't have any health problems that could be preventing your weight loss. This can be frustrating, but stick with it, stay positive, and stay in the game. When the keto diet is done correctly, it is one of the best ways to lose weight.

Chapter 9 How Keto Diet Affects 50 Old Women

Women who are looking for a quick and effective way to shed excess weight, get high blood sugar levels under control, reduce overall inflammations, and improve physical and mental energy will do their best by following a ketogenic diet plan. But there are special considerations women must take into account when they are beginning the keto diet.

All women know it is much more difficult for women to lose weight than it is for men to lose weight. A woman will live on a starvation level diet and exercise like a triathlete and only lose five pounds. A man will stop putting dressing on his salad and will lose twenty pounds. It just is not fair. But we have the fact that we are women to blame. Women naturally have more standing between them and weight loss than men do.

The mere fact that we are women is the largest single contributor to the reason we find it difficult to lose weight. Since our bodies always think they need to be prepared for the possibility of pregnancy women will naturally have more body fat and less mass in our muscles than men will. Muscle cells burn more calories than fat cells do. So because we are women we will always lose weight more slowly than men will.

Being in menopause will also cause women to add more pounds to their bodies, especially in the lower half of the body. After menopause a woman's metabolism naturally slows down. Your hormones levels will decrease. These two factors alone will cause weight gain in the post-menopausal woman.

Women are a direct product of their hormones. Men also have hormones but not the ones like we have that regulate every function in our bodies. And the hormones in women will fluctuate around their everyday habits like lack of sleep, poor eating habits, and menstrual cycles. These hormones cause women to crave sweets around the time their periods occur. These cravings will wreck any diet plan. Staying true to the keto plan is challenging at this time because of the intense craving for sweets and carbs. Also having your period will often make you feel and look bloated because of the water your body holds onto during this time. And having cramps make you more likely to reach for a bag of cookies than a plate of steak and salad.

Because we are women we may experience challenges on the keto diet that men will not face because they are men. One of these challenges is having weight loss plateau or even experiencing weight gain. This can happen because of the influence of hormones on weight loss in women. If this happens you will want to increase your consumption of good fats like ghee, butter, eggs, coconut oil, beef, avocados, and olive oil. Any food that is cooked or prepared using oil must be prepared in olive oil or avocado oil.

You can also use MCT oil. MCT stands for medium chain triglycerides. This is a form of fatty acid that is saturated and has many health benefits. MCT can help with many body functions from weight loss to improved brain function. MCTs are mostly missing from the typical American diet because we have been told that saturated fats are harmful to the body, and as a group they are. But certain saturated fats, like MCTs, are actually beneficial to the body, especially when they come from good foods like beef or coconut oil. They are easier to digest than most other saturated fats and may help improve heart and brain function and prevent obesity.

Many women on a keto diet will struggle with imbalances in their hormones. On the keto diet you do not rely on lowered calories to lose weight but on foods effect on your hormones. So when women begin the keto diet any issues they are already having with their hormones will be brought to attention and may cause the woman to give up before she really begins. Always remember that the keto diet is responsible for cleansing the system first so that the body can easily respond to the wonderful affects a keto diet has to offer.

Do not try to work toward the lean body that many men sport. It is best for overall function that women stay at twenty two to twenty six percent body fat. Our hormones will function best in this range and we can't possible function without our hormones. Women who are very lean, like gymnasts and extreme athletes, will find their hormones no longer function or function at a less than optimal rate. And remember that ideal weight may not be the right weight for you.

Many women find that they perform their best when they are at their happy weight. If you find yourself fighting with yourself to lose the last few pounds you think you need to lose in order to have the perfect body then it may not be worth it. The struggle will affect your hormone function. Carefully observing the keto diet will allow time for your hormones to stabilize and regulate themselves back to their pre-obesity normal function.

Like any other diet plan the keto diet will work better if you are active. Regular exercise will allow the body to strengthen and tone muscles and will help to work off excess fat reserves. But exercise requires energy to accomplish. If you restrict your carb intake too much you might not have the energy needed to be physically able to make it all the way through the day and still be able to maintain an exercise routine. You might need to add in more carbs to your diet through the practice of carb cycling.

As a woman you know that sometimes your emotions get the better of you. This is true with your body, as you well know, and can be a major reason why women find it extremely difficult at times to lose weight the way they want to lose weight. We have been led to believe that not only can we do it all but that we must do it all. This gives many women unnecessary levels of pressure and can cause them to engage in emotional eating. Some women might have lowered feelings of self-worth and may not feel they are entitled to the benefits of the keto diet, and turning to food relieves the feelings of inadequacy that we try to hide from the world.

When you engage in the same activity for a long period of time it becomes a habit. When you reach for the bag of potato chips or the tub of ice cream whenever you are angry, upset, or depressed, then your brain will eventually tell you to reach for food whenever you feel an emotion that you don't want to deal with. Food acts as a security blanket against the world outside. It may be necessary to address any extreme emotional issues you are having before you begin the keto diet, so that you are better assured of success.

The basic act of staying on the keto diet can be very challenging for some women. Many women see beginning a new diet to lose weight as a punishment for being overweight. It may be worthwhile for you to work at changing the set of your mind if you are feeling this way. You may need to remind yourself daily that the keto diet is not a punishment but a blessing for your body. Tell yourself that you are not denying yourself certain foods because you can't eat them, but because you do not like the way those foods make your body feel. Don't watch other people eating their high carb diet and pity yourself. Instead, feel sorry for the people who have trapped themselves in a high calorie diet and are not experiencing the benefits that you are experiencing.

And for the first thirty days cut out all sweeteners, even the non-sugar ones that are allowed on the keto diet. While they may make food taste better they also remind your brain that it needs sweet foods when it really doesn't. Cutting them out for at least thirty days will break the cycle that your body has fallen into and will cut the cravings for sweets in your diet.

It is very possible for women to be successful on the keto diet if they are prepared to follow a few simple adjustment that will make the diet look differently than your male partner might be eating but that will make you successful in the long run.

During the first one or two weeks you will need to consume extra fat than a man might need to. Doing this will have three important effects on your body. First it will cause your mitochondria to intensify their acceptance of your new way of finding energy. Mitochondria are tiny organisms that are found in cells and are responsible for using the fuel that insulin brings to the cell for fuel for the cell. Increasing your fat intake will also help make sure you are getting enough calories in your daily diet. This is important because if your body thinks you are starving it will begin to conserve calories and you will stop losing weight.

The third benefit from eating more fat, and perhaps the most important, is the psychological boost you will get from seeing that you can eat more fat and still lose weight and feel good. It will also reset your mindset that you previously might have held against fat. For so long we have been told that low fat is the only way to lose weight. But an absence of dietary fat will lead to overeating and binge eating out of a feeling of deprivation. When you begin the diet by allowing yourself to eat a lot, or too much in your mind, fat, then you swing the pendulum around to the other side of the fat scale where it properly belongs. You teach yourself that fat can be good for you. Increasing the extra intake of fats should not last beyond the second week of the diet. Your body will improve its abilities to create and burn ketones and body fat, and then you will begin using your own body fat for fuel and you can begin to lower your reliance on dietary fat a little bit so that you will begin to lose weight.

The keto diet is naturally lower in calories if you follow the recommended levels of food intake. It is not necessary to try to restrict your intake of calories even further. All you need to do is to eat only until you are full and not one bite more. Besides losing weight the aim of the keto diet is to retrain your body on how to work properly. You will need to learn to trust your body and the signals it send out to be able to readjust to a proper way of eating. So don't feel you need to consume every bite on your plate. If having leftovers bothers you then make just one portion for each person to consume and no more. Left to its own devices your body systems will properly regulate themselves and this includes the intake of food. Give the keto diet a chance to work properly.

The major point of the keto diet is to help your body burn fat. Fasting will also help you burn fat. It is often beneficial to combine fasting with the keto diet to gain the best possible benefits from your new lifestyle and the changes you have made.

Do not feel you always need to be so strict with yourself by denying yourself any and every little treat. Stick to the keto diet as closely as possible for the first four weeks, and then after that give yourself permission to fail every once in a while. After you make it through the first four weeks you have arrived. Your body is now a true fat burning machine. The mitochondria in your cells have accepted the fact that their energy now comes from fat instead of sugar. So enjoying that one little cookie with your child is not going to completely derail your diet and all your success. The idea here is to teach the body that it is able to cheat a little and get right back on track without issue. It is the ability to live in the real world and live like a 'normal' person. You will find that you will bounce right back from your little moment of enjoyment. But don't ever look at it as cheating. It is just a way to live normally. You will be fine.

While it is fine to eventually give yourself a little treat it is important to watch out for the possibility for carbs to creep back into your diet. If you have been doing well and suddenly find your weight loss has stalled examine the things you have been eating. It is very easy for carbs to creep back into your diet especially in the form of nuts, fruits, condiments, and sauces. It is very easy to consume too many carbs simply by eating a few extra nuts as a snack or adding too much sauce to something you are eating.

And do not fall into the trap of restricting your protein. Protein is often the first food to fall off the plate when women don't experience rapid weight loss on the keto diet. Multiple internet searches will recommend dropping your intake of protein to a level comparable to your intake of carbs. Doing that will mean that you will be living on nothing but fat and you might even begin to gain weight. Too much protein in the diet can get in the way of ketosis, but there is such a thing as not getting enough protein in your diet. And women generally eat less protein than men do anyway. Throwing your body into ketosis rapidly is meaningless if your body is consuming its own muscle mass to survive. And that is exactly what it will do. The body needs a certain amount of protein intake to survive. If you do not consume enough protein for the body's process it will turn to its own muscles for protein. You will lose muscle mass and eventually you will begin to gain weight.

While making sure you are eating enough protein it might be a good idea to add a bit of weight training to your daily routine. Weight training will help you build muscles mass and that will help you increase the rate at which your metabolism works. A faster metabolism will burn fat faster, and muscle mass will burn more calories than fat will. Your weight lifting does not need to be an immense undertaking. Five to ten minutes two or three times a week will be enough in the beginning. The key is to lift a weight that is heavy enough to cause muscle failure. This just means that after lifting the weight for ten or fifteen times, called reps, you are physically unable to lift the weight one more time. This is called muscle failure and it is necessary to be able to build muscles. The muscle will tear slightly and will release toxins. When the muscle heals it will be stronger and larger. Don't worry; you won't grow big Popeye-type muscles.

You must make sure you are getting enough sleep. I know it is common for women to stay up late or get up early in order to 'get more done' but this will work against you. You are straining your body in ways it has not strained in a long time. It needs a proper amount of rest in order to rebuild itself and prepare for the next day. And during the first two to three weeks, as your body is going into ketosis, you will feel sleepier and more tired than ever before, except maybe during pregnancy. This period will pass eventually but in the meantime give your body what it really needs in the form of seven to nine hours of sleep each night.

Following a keto diet can bring numerous benefits to the body, but it must be done the right way. Women have less room for making mistakes on the diet than men do. You will need to find the keto plan that works best for you and be prepared to follow it. No one version is right for everyone; even men follow different versions of the keto diet. It is definitely a learning process to find the combination of foods that will cause you to lose weight and feel your best. Be patient and listen to your body and you will find that you will be successful.

Chapter 10 Benefits Of Keto Diet For Women Over

The keto diet has become so popular in recent years because of the success people have noticed. Not only have they managed to lose weight, but scientific studies show that the keto diet can help you improve your health in many others. As when starting any new diet or exercise routine, there may seem to be some disadvantages so we will go over those for the keto diet as well. But most people agree that the benefits outweigh the adjustment period!

Benefits

Losing weight! For most people, this is the first and foremost benefit of switching to keto! Their previous diet method may have stalled for them or they were starting to notice weight creeping back on. With keto, studies have shown that people have been able to follow this diet and relay fewer hunger pangs and suppressed appetite while losing weight at the same time! You are minimizing your carbohydrate intake which means less blood sugar spikes. Often, those fluctuations in blood sugar levels are what make you feel more hungry and prone to snacking in between meals. Instead, by guiding the body towards ketosis, you are eating a more fulfilling diet of fat and protein and harnessing energy from ketone molecules instead of glucose. Studies show that low carb diets are very effective in reducing visceral fat (the type of fat you commonly see around the abdomen that increases as you become overweight and obese). This reduces your risk of obesity and improves your health in the long run.

Decreases the risk of Type 2 diabetes. As we mentioned in the previous chapter, the problem with carbohydrates is how unstable they make blood sugar levels. This can be very dangerous for people who have diabetes or are considered pre-diabetic due to unstable blood sugar levels or family history. Keto is a great option because of the minimal intake of carbohydrates it requires. Instead, you are harnessing the majority of your calories from fat or protein which will not cause blood sugar spikes and ultimately put less pressure on the pancreas to secrete insulin. Many studies have found that diabetes patients who followed the keto diet lost more weight and ultimately reduced their fasting glucose levels. This is great news for patients who have unstable blood sugar levels or are hoping to avoid or reduce their diabetes medication intake.

Improve cardiovascular risk symptoms to overall lower your chances of having heart disease. Most people assume that following keto that is so high in fat content has to increase your risk of coronary heart disease or heart attack. But the research proves otherwise! Research shows that switching to keto can lower your blood pressure, increase your HDL good cholesterol, and reduce your triglyceride fatty acid levels. That's because the fat you are consuming on keto are healthy and high-quality fats so they tend to reverse many unhealthy symptoms of heart disease. They boost your "good" HDL cholesterol numbers and decrease your "bad" LDL cholesterol numbers. It also decreases the level of triglyceride fatty acids in the bloodstream. A high level of these can lead to stroke, heart attack, or premature death. And what are high levels of fatty acids linked to? High consumption of carbohydrates. With the keto diet, you are drastically cutting your intake of carbohydrates to improve fatty acid levels and improve other risk factors. A 2018 study on the keto diet found that it can improve as many as 22 out of 26 risk factors for cardiovascular heart disease! These factors can be very important to some people, especially those who have a history of heart disease in their family.

Increases the body's energy levels. We compared briefly about the difference between the glucose molecules synthesized from a high carbohydrates intake versus ketones produced on the keto diet. Ketones are made by the liver and use fat molecules you already have stored. This makes them much more energy-rich and a lasting source of fuel compared to glucose, a simple sugar molecule. These ketones can give you a burst of energy physically as well as mentally allow you to have greater focus, clarity, and attention to detail.

Decreases inflammation in the body. Inflammation on its own is a natural response by the body's immune system, but when it becomes uncontrollable, it can lead to an array of health problems, some severe, some minor. The many health concerns include acne, autoimmune conditions, arthritis, psoriasis, irritable bowel syndrome, and even acne and eczema. Often, removing sugars and carbohydrates from your diet can help patients of these diseases avoid flare-ups - and the good news is keto does just that! A 2008 research study found that keto decreased a blood marker linked to high inflammation in the body by nearly 40%. This is great news for people who may suffer from an inflammatory disease and are willing to change their diet to hopefully see improvement.

Increases your mental functioning level. Like we elaborated earlier, the energy-rich ketones can boost the body's physical and mental levels of alertness. Research has shown that keto is a much better energy source for the brain than simple sugar glucose molecules are. With nearly 75% of your diet coming from healthy fats, the brain's neural cells and mitochondria have a better source of energy to be able to function at the highest level. Some studies have tested patients on the keto diet and found they had higher cognitive functioning, better memory recall, and were less susceptible to memory loss. The keto diet can even decrease the occurrence of migraines which can be very detrimental to patients.

Decreases risk of diseases like Alzheimer's, Parkinson's, and epilepsy. The keto diet was actually created in the 1920s as a way to combat epilepsy in children. From there, research has found that keto can improve your cognitive functioning level and protect brain cells from injury or damage. This is very good to reduce the risk of neurodegenerative disease which begins in the brain due to neural cells mutating and functioning with damaged parts or lower than peak optimal functioning. Studies have found that following keto can improve the mental functioning of patients who suffer from diseases like Alzheimer's or Parkinson's. These neurodegenerative diseases sadly have no cure, but the keto diet could improve symptoms as they progress. Researchers believe that is due to cutting out carbs from your diet which reduces the occurrence of blood sugar spikes that the body's neural cells have to continually adjust to.

Can regulate hormones in women who have PCOS (polycystic ovary syndrome) and PMS (pre-menstrual syndrome). Women who have PCOS suffer from infertility which can be very heartbreaking for young couples trying to start a family. There is no cure for this condition, but it is believed that it is related to many similar diabetic symptoms like obesity and high insulin levels. This causes the body to produce more sex hormones which can lead to infertility. The keto diet has become a popular method to try and regulate insulin and hormone levels and could increase a woman's chances of getting pregnant.

Disadvantages

Your body will have an adjustment period. It depends from person to person on how many days that will be, but when you start any new diet or exercise routine, your body has to adjust to the new normal. With the keto diet, you are drastically cutting your carbohydrates intake, so the body has to adjust to that. You may feel slow, weak, fatigued, and like you are not thinking as quick or fast as you used to. It just means your body is adjusting to keto and once this adjustment period is done, you will see the weight loss results you anticipated.

If you are an athlete, you may need more carbohydrates. If you still want to try keto as an athlete, it's important you talk to your nutritionist or trainer to see how the diet can be tweaked for you. Most athletes require a greater intake of carbs than the keto diet requires which means they may have to up their intake in order to assure they have the energy for their training sessions. High endurance sports (like rugby or soccer) and heavy weightlifting do require a greater intake of carbohydrates. If you're an athlete wanting to follow keto and gain the health benefits, it's important you first talk to your trainer before making any changes to your diet.

You have to carefully count your daily macros! For beginners, this can be tough, and even people already on keto can become lazy about this. People are often used to eating what they want without worrying about just how many grams of protein or carbs it contains. With keto, you have to be meticulous about counting your intake to ensure you are maintaining the necessary keto breakdown (75% fat, 20% protein, ~5% carbs). The closer you stick to this, the better results you will see regarding weight loss and other health benefits. If your weight loss has stalled or you're not feeling as energetic as you hoped, it could be because your macros are off. Find a free calorie counting app that and be sure you look at the ingredients of everything you're eating and cooking.

Chapter 11 Tips And Trick For Women Over 50

The ultimate objective of a ketogenic diet is to make your body enter into a specific metabolic state known as ketosis. As mentioned earlier, when your body depletes the entire glycogen stores it turns to the fat stores to produce ketones which in turn give energy to the cells in your body. This means, your body's energy source is no more glucose but the ketones.

But there seems to be a problem here – many people who start with the ketogenic diet have a problem in entering into the ketosis state or staying in the ketosis state after they get in! They often push themselves out of the ketosis state. You can overcome this if you avoid the mistakes that amateurs make.

Don't be scared of fat

If you want to lose your extra fat then you will have to take in more fat. Does it sound silly? Well, not if you have heard this – "You have to spend money to make money!"

Keto applies a similar logic – your body needs more dietary fat and extremely less dietary carbs to get into ketosis. If you want to change your body to a fat-burning machine, then you should first deprive it of carbs (primary energy source: glycogen – stored glucose). When you do that, your body senses that it has not been getting enough glucose through food and so it starts to use the stored glucose (glycogen). Once it completely exhausts the reserve, it begins to look for an alternate energy source.

Your body targets the stored body fat and breaks it down into fatty acids. These fatty acids produce ketones. When this happens, your body enters into an entirely new metabolic state – ketosis! So, eating more healthy fats is actually going to help you get rid of all the water weight and extra flab. Therefore, you can consume butter and cheese.

Water is important

You need to consistently drink enough water all through the day to keep your body hydrated. The generic advice given by the medical experts is – you need to drink at least one gallon of water every day to help your body's organ to function properly and do its respective job!

It might be hard if you are a working professional but my advice to you is to keep a bottle of clean drinking water next to your workplace. Keep sipping it as often as possible. When you have water near you, you naturally tend to drink more water than you normally do!

You might have to make frequent visits to the restroom but that is fine, as over a period of time your body will get used to your new drinking routine and handle things accordingly.

Get Salty

If you are a first-time keto dieter, you might experience some of the keto flu symptoms. Constant headaches, fatigue, feeling feverish, etc. – but you do not need to worry, you get these symptoms because your body is trying to adapt to a new routine. It is definitely possible to prevent these flu-like symptoms!

You are losing more electrolytes as you are eating real, wholesome food and drinking loads of water. No junk stuff and artificial preservatives are getting into your body. There is a bit of cleansing activity happening in your body – so you have to help your body by refilling the lost electrolytes.

How do you do it? The simplest way to do it is by adding salt (sodium) into your body. You can mix a teaspoon of salt to your drinking water and have it once a day. You can also add sriracha or chili garlic sauce to your food as they have sodium. You can add a bit more salt while you are giving extra seasoning to your salads or other dishes.

There is another benefit in consuming more salt – your body will be able to retain water effortlessly thereby reducing your trips to the restroom!

Dairy is good but don't go overboard

The protocol of the ketogenic diet is to include a large amount of high-fat food items and the most commonly used high-fat food source is – full-fat dairy.

The issue here is, when you consume too much dairy (more than the required calorie amount), you suddenly begin to realize that you have reached a plateau. At this stage, you do not lose any more weight.

Why? The theory here is – if you need to lose weight, you need to put your body into a calorie deficit mode i.e. give it fewer calories.

For instance – if your body is burning around 1500 calories daily and you consume 1000 calories, now your body needs to find the remaining 500 calories to burn. When you are in keto, you give that to your body in the form of fat. Coming back to our dairy products – since most dairy items are rich in calories, it is quite natural for you to over-eat resulting in calorie overload. This means – you do not allow your body to burn the extra fat for more energy as you are already feeding it with the required fat.

It is good to add a good amount of mozzarella to your meals but do not eat the entire block of mozzarella in one go.

Know your WHY factor

The important part of any diet is – you should know WHY you are doing it. Are you practicing a particular diet because you want to look good? Or are you doing it to improve your overall health? Whatever the reason is you need to fix it strong in your mind. 99 percent of your diet's success lies in your psychology – your mental capacity should be strong! You need to be sure of why you are doing it and believe that it will work!

You might often get tempted to consume things that will push you out of ketosis. You need to think about your WHY during those times. Your goal, your objective is important! It is okay if you cheat once, do not crib over it. Think positive – ask yourself the question, why should I not get back on track? I can get back on the board and reach my destination soon.

The WHY should motivate you and push you forward to reach your goal. It has a real strong emotion!

Too much protein isn't good

This is another reason for your body to go out of ketosis state. Since you can include meat in your diet, there are times that you often tend to over-eat the meat dishes. Too much protein can produce glucose through the gluconeogenesis process. The body first converts excess protein to glycogen, and converts the glycogen into fat.

Adding chicken breast to your diet routine is good but eating a whole bucket of the chicken fry is probably not going to do any good for your keto diet. Remember to take note of your daily macros to avoid such instances. Otherwise, buy less meat while you go for your grocery shopping!

Stop snacking often

Too much snacking can knock you out of ketosis as it can spike up your blood sugar levels. The good thing with a keto diet is since you include a good amount of high fat to your food you get to feel more satiated. So your temptation to have snacks reduces especially when you have included more fiber to your food platter.

A handful of almonds for energy is good but a bowl of cashews is not! The best way to reduce too much snacking is – to prepare your meal much in advance of your eating time so that you do not indulge in snacking as you cook your meal.

No more habit-eating

Gaining better control over your appetite is one of the best things about the keto diet. Most people listen to their stomach growl and walk toward the refrigerator or pantry in search of something to eat. You should give that habit up to avoid giving into your cravings. You might not experience these things after 2 to 3 weeks of keto dieting.

But few people might experience a hiccup here – since you are eating in a specific way for some time, you get accustomed to that habit. For instance, you might be used to eating something after every three hours and this habit eating will now take you to the refrigerator even when you are not hungry. You need to consciously work toward switching off your mind to this habit. The best way to achieve this is by planning your meals much earlier – meal plan plays an important role in the keto diet.

Sleep is essential

If you are not giving your mind and body the much-required rest, your system is going to face difficulty in doing things it is supposed to do. Good quality sleep is important to control your stress, give rest to your organs and to make you feel energetic the following day.

Eight hours of sleep is mandatory and thankfully following a well-planned keto diet will give you the required sleep without any issues. But if you are a party animal, do not blame me!

Stress management

Over-stressing yourself is going to increase the cortisol levels in your body. What is cortisol? The stress hormone increases your blood sugar level hindering your weight-loss plan.

When your body experiences a consecutive rise and fall in your blood sugar levels, it sends a confusing signal to your brain. Your brain naturally assumes that it is time to refill the glycogen reserve and so it sends you a signal by telling that it needs carbs now! Your body craves for sugar when it is under stress. This is the survival mechanism of the body! If you want to have a successful keto journey, then you need to work on your stress management.

Don't eat the same meal every time

You need to mix up your meals or else you will get bored too soon. There are so many keto-friendly recipes out there and all you need to do is choose the ones that are best for you. You can also discover your own new recipes by adding in your touch of culinary expertise. Add some low-carb veggies to your usual keto meal and spice it up with herbs and condiments.

When there are numerous options available why would you want to eat the same lunch and dinner for the entire month? Unleash your creativity and turn your kitchen into an experimentation lab!

No cheat days

There are few diets which offer you cheat days so that you can wolf down all your favorite stuff on that one day. But beware – there are no cheat days in keto. This is a strict diet routine and you need to adhere to its protocols if you want to achieve your goal weight. If you feel like having a sponge cake or milk chocolate, make a fat bomb and have it.

Keto offers you a substitute for almost everything. Be aware of your mistakes and make preparations accordingly. It is crucial to plan your meals to avoid these commonly repetitive mistakes. Once you get into ketosis, it is not that easy to come out of it but it is not easy to stay on it either!

Quick tips you can follow

Keto is a simple, straightforward diet routine but you need to know the basics before you jump into it.

- How do you cook easy keto meals?

- I have been avoiding fats all these years, how do I get it back to my diet?

- My work routine often forces me to eat out once in a week. How do I manage to stay on keto then?

- How do I start my day on a keto diet?

These common questions might pop up when you are following the diet for the first time. It is quite simple to get started with keto – no complications at all!

- You can consume eggs in any form; however, it is best to add more coconut oil, olive oil and butter while preparing the eggs.

- You do not necessarily need to start your day with a mandatory breakfast. No, it is not really the important meal of the day – breaking the fast (breakfast) is important. So if you are not hungry in the morning, you do not need to eat for the sake of eating. Drink loads of water, have a cup of herbal tea or a cup of coffee. You often experience reduced hunger when you are on keto, so skipping a meal is fine!

- If you are someone who wakes up with a grumbling stomach every morning, not to worry there are tons of easy-to-make breakfast recipes available. You can get hold of a few in this book too!

- Plan your main meals (lunch and dinner) much ahead of time. A simple main course made of meat or fish accompanied by a vegetable side or a salad. Or a super nutritious vegetable main with a healthy smoothie should do the magic!

- If you feel constantly hungry when you start the keto diet, eat more fat and fiber-rich food – eggs, leafy greens, cruciferous veggies, etc.

- If you are out at an official dinner party or a get-together with your friends, replace your pasta or bread with veggie mains + olive oil or butter.

- Go for a fish-based dish or replace the high-carb food with extra mixed vegetables. Try the egg-based meals – scrambled eggs, omelet, fried eggs, etc.

- Choose the burgers without buns and replace your French fries with veggies and add a bit of cheese or guacamole to it

- Mexican dishes offer extra salsa, cheese and sour cream

- Choose berries with cream, mixed cheese board as your dessert option

Chapter 12 The Best Keto Diet Foods For Dieting After 50 Years Old

The next step is to restock your pantry, fridge and freezer. It's time to go shopping for delicious, keto-friendly foods that will help you lose weight, become healthier, and feel and look great.

As in all things, its best to start off simple. Stock up on the basics and you'll always be ready to prepare healthy, keto-friendly meals and snacks.

THE BASICS

Be sure to pick up these basics first thing.

- Water, coffee, and tea

- All spices and herbs (check the labels for added sugars!)

- Sweeteners, including Stevia and erythritol and monk fruit sweetener

- Lemon and lime juice

- Low-carb condiments such as mayonnaise, mustard, pesto, and sriracha

- Broths (chicken, beef, bone)

• Pickled and fermented foods like pickles, kimchi, and sauerkraut

• Nuts and seeds: including macadamia nuts, pecans, almonds, walnuts, hazelnuts, pine nuts, flaxseed, chia seeds, and pumpkin seeds.

Once you've gotten the basics, it time to concentrate on those items that will make up the majority of your menus.

MEATS

Any type of meat is acceptable for the keto diet. Enjoy chicken, beef, lamb, pork, turkey, etc. A lot of people will tell you to purchase grass-fed/organic meats if they are available, but this isn't necessary and it can impact your budget. Just be sure to get as fresh as possible and you'll be fine. One of the perks about the keto diet is that it is more than acceptable to eat the fat and skin on the chicken. Fish and seafood have a prominent place in the keto diet! Eggs also hold an important place here.

VEGATABLES

Avoid all types of potatoes, yams, corn, and legumes like beans, lentils, and peas. You can eat all non-starchy veggies including broccoli, spinach, asparagus, mushrooms, cucumbers, lettuce, onions, peppers, brussels sprouts, zucchini, eggplant, olives, yellow squash and cauliflower. Tomatoes are also acceptable in limited quantities because they do have a higher carb count.

FRUITS

Most fruits are off limits on the keto diet due to the high levels of sugars they contain. A Single banana for example, has around 25 grams of carbohydrates! However, you may eat small amounts of berries every day such as strawberries, raspberries, blackberries, and blueberries. Lemon and lime juices are great for adding flavor to your meals. Avocados are also low in carbs and full of healthy fat.

DAIRY

Always eat full-fat dairy like butter, sour cream, heavy whipping cream, cheese, cream cheese, and unsweetened yogurt. Avoid milk and skim milk, as well as sweetened yogurts as they contain great amounts of sugar. Although technically not dairy, you can enjoy unsweetened almond and coconut milks as well.

FATS AND OILS

Avocado oil, olive oil, butter, lard, and bacon fat are great for cooking as well as general consumption. Avocado oil has a high smoke point (it does not burn or smoke until it reaches 550 F), which is ideal for searing meats and frying in a wok.

Add beef and chicken bouillon to the list as well. Make sure the bouillon cubes have at least 1 gram of sodium. Why? When carbs are cut, we rapidly deplete our store of glycogen (what carbohydrates are converted into when we eat them). For every gram of glycogen we lose, we lose 3 grams of water. Adding the bouillon will help prevent dehydration and improve the way you feel on the diet. Water isn't enough on keto: you need enough sodium as well.

YOUR KITCHEN

There are certain items that could make your life much simpler in the kitchen, but these are definitely not must-haves. If you feel that they would benefit your diet plan, and you have the money to spare, then following is a list of kitchen items that would be useful.

FOOD SCALE

A must have for anyone serious about weight loss. A food scale comes in quite handy for measuring your foods to make sure you are counting your macros and portions correctly. You can measure solids, or liquid food stuffs and be sure to get the perfect amount every time. It's not as easy to "guesstimate", but it can be done. A food scale used in conjunction with a carb counting app will help to ensure you hit your weight loss goals more quickly.

FOOD PROCESSOR

A food processor has more power than a typical blender when it's time to blend foods together for making sauces, or simply chopping down tough vegetables like cauliflower and broccoli. The food processor can also be used for kneading, making batters, slicing, chopping, cutting, shredding, grinding, or mincing. They can perform the task at hand with high efficiency in no time at all.

SPIRALIZER

Spiralizers make vegetables into noodles or ribbons within seconds. Vegetables like zucchini are naturally gluten-free, light in calories, carbs, and sugars which make them a great substitute for flour-based pastas. By spiralizing, you're naturally eating more vegetables without even noticing! Eating a bowl full of spiralized veggies will fool your taste buds into believing that you're enjoying your favorite pasta dishes while your waistline realizes the benefits of a healthy eating habit.

ELECTRIC HAND MIXER

Perhaps the best advantage of an electric hand mixer is the cost. Much less expensive than a stand mixer, the hand mixer also takes up less space in the kitchen. It's perfect for small jobs like blending or mixing cream cheese dishes, beating egg whites and whipping cream.

If you've ever had to mix egg whites by hand, your arm muscles will thank you for investing in an electric hand mixer!

CAST IRON PANS

If you own cast iron pots and pans, now's the time to get them out. Cooking in cast iron is much healthier than using Teflon coated or other chemical treated pans, and they last pretty much forever. However, if you don't presently own these, do not by any means feel like you must go out and buy them! Whatever you currently have in the way of pots and pans is perfectly acceptable. Remember, the goal is to learn to cook and eat healthy, not to break the bank!

Chapter 13 Best Exercises To Lose Weight After 50 Years Old

When people picture themselves making better life choices, they often picture themselves eating better and then following this up with a lot of cardio and sit-ups. This, of course, can be a part of the ketogenic diet, but first, you need to change many of the ideas you probably have over exercise and dieting.

When the image of someone "dieting" springs to a person's mind, they often think of someone who is eating much less than average and following up this pitiful meal by working out for an hour. This model is not only unsustainable but ridiculous. We've already covered that the keto diet can be full of rich, enjoyable meals that will fuel your body and make you feel good. Exercise can be equally enriching.

Just in case you don't know, exercise is primarily fueled by glucose. When glucose is stored as glycogen, it is the glycogen stores that get burned when you do strenuous exercise. So, you may be wondering how exercising works on the keto diet, considering that you're switching your body over to burning fat.

Some people may read the fact that exercise burns glucose and think that exercise is impossible. Or that they shouldn't bother.

To be clear: you can get by without worrying about exercise. The majority of our health comes from what we eat, and as long as you're moving around a lot during the day in the form of walking and standing, you should be fine. Although, exercise does have its health benefits. It helps makes our bones stronger, enhances muscle growth and sustainability, and is good for the heart. So, implementing even just a light exercise routine is very beneficial.

There are four kinds of exercise you can do:

Aerobic: this is what is commonly known as cardio and is anything that's high intensity and lasts for over three minutes. It predominantly uses carbs as an energy source.

Anaerobic Exercise: this is what people consider interval training. It requires shorter bursts of energy, and carbs are once again its primary source of energy. Think of weight training or high cardio interval training.

Flexibility: this is anything that stretches your body. Think yoga, or after workout stretches. This kind of exercise is great for your joints, improving your muscle range of motion, and helps prevent injuries.

Stability: think balancing exercises and core training. It improves alignment, strengthens muscles, and helps control movements.

What energy is burned really depends on the intensity of your workout, but the gist of it is this:

Low-intensity: fat is used as energy

High-intensity: glycogen is used as energy

Pretty simple, right?

However, that does mean that you need to consume more carbs if you do more high-intensity workouts. It goes back to the fact that the more you work out, the more carbs you need. You're going to have to adjust the carbs based on your lifestyle.

If you exercise more than three times a week, consider looking into a different kind of ketogenic diet, specifically the Targeted Keto Diet.

We already talked a bit about it before, but the idea is that you eat all your carbs around the time you work out. Eat 15 g to 30 g of carbs right before and right after. This gives your muscles glycogen to help your muscles recover, and any extra glucose will be burned away by the workout.

For the first few weeks of the keto diet, exercise will be pretty hard on your body. This means that for this time, you're going to have to take it easy, like with walks and light yoga. The longer your body gets used to burning fats for energy, the better you will feel. You will find your exercise performance will increase after a few weeks.

In the beginning, focus on the diet first, rather than the exercise. Feeding your body with the proper nutrients it needs and letting it adapt to the different fuel source is more important, at first. After your body gets adjusted, you will find it much easier.

Chapter 14 Recipes

Breakfast

Eggs and Ham

Preparation **Time**: 25 minutes

Servings: 4

Ingredients:

4 eggs

10 ham slices

4 tbsp. scallions

A pinch of black pepper

A pinch of sweet paprika

1 tbsp. melted ghee

Directions:

Grease a muffin pan with melted ghee.

Divide ham slicesin each muffin mold to form your cups. In a bowl; mix eggs with scallions, pepper and paprika and whisk well.

Divide this mix on top of ham, introduce your ham cups in the oven at 400 °F and bake for 15 minutes. Leave cups to cool down before dividing on plates and serving.

Nutrition Values: Calories: 250; Fat: 10g; Fiber: 3g; Carbs: 6g; Protein: 12g

Italian Style Eggs

Preparation **Time**: 25 minutes

Servings: 1

Ingredients:

2 eggs

1/4 tsp. rosemary; dried

1/2 cup cherry tomatoes halved

1½ cups kale; chopped

1/2 tsp. coconut oil

3 tbsp. water

1 tsp. balsamic vinegar

1/4 avocado; peeled and chopped

Directions:

Heat up a pan with the oil over medium high heat, add water, kale, rosemary and tomatoes, stir; cover and cook for 4 minutes.

Uncover pan, stir again and add eggs.

Stir and scramble eggs for 3 minutes.

Add vinegar, stir everything and transfer to a serving plate. Top with chopped avocado and serve.

Nutrition Values: Calories: 185; Fat: 10g; Fiber: 1g; Carbs: 6g; Protein: 7g

Orange and Dates Granola

Preparation **Time**: 25 minutes

Servings: 6

Ingredients:

5 oz. dates; soaked in hot water

1/2 cup pumpkin seeds

Juice from 1 orange

Grated rind of 1/2 orange

1 cup desiccated coconut

1/2 cup silvered almonds

1/2 cup linseeds

1/2 cup sesame seeds

Almond milk for serving

Directions:

In a bowl; mix almonds with orange rind, orange juice, linseeds, coconut, pumpkin and sesame seeds and stir well.

Drain dates, add them to your food processor and blend well. Add this paste to almonds mix and stir well again.

Spread this on a lined baking sheet, introduce in the oven at 350 °F and bake for 15 minutes, stirring every 4 minutes.

Take granola out of the oven, leave aside to cool down a bit and then serve with almond milk.

Nutrition Values: Calories: 208g; Protein: 6g; Fiber: 5; Fat: 9; Sugar: 0

Bacon Muffins

Preparation **Time**: 40 minutes

Servings: 4

Ingredients:

4 oz. bacon slices

3 garlic cloves; minced

1 small yellow onion; chopped

1 zucchini; thinly sliced

A handful spinach; torn

6 canned and pickled artichoke hearts; chopped

8 eggs

1/4 tsp. paprika

A pinch of black pepper

A pinch of cayenne pepper

1/4 cup coconut cream

Directions:

Heat up a pan over medium high heat, add bacon, stir; cook until it's crispy, transfer to paper towels, drain grease and leave aside for now.

Heat up the same pan over medium heat again, add garlic and onion, stir and cook for 4 minutes.

In a bowl; mix eggs with coconut cream, onions, garlic, paprika, black pepper and cayenne and whisk well.

Add spinach, zucchini and artichoke pieces and stir everything.

Divide crispy bacon slices in a muffin pan, add eggs mixture on top, introduce your muffins in the oven and bake at 400 °F for 20 minutes. Leave them to cool down before serving them for breakfast.

Nutrition Values: Calories: 270; Fat: 12g; Fiber: 4g; Carbs: 6g; Protein: 12g

Parsley and Pear Smoothie

Preparation **Time**: 5 minutes

Servings: 6

Ingredients:

1 apple pear; chopped

1 bunch parsley; roughly chopped

1 small avocado; stoned and peeled

1 pear; peeled and chopped

1 green apple; chopped

1 Granny Smith apple; chopped

6 bananas; peeled and roughly chopped

2 plums; stoned

1 cup ice

1 cup water

Directions:

In your kitchen blender, mix parsley with avocado, apple pear, pear, green apple, Granny Smith apple, plums and bananas and blend very well.

Add ice and water and blend again very well. Transfer to tall glasses and serve right away.

Nutrition Values: Calories: 208g; Carbs: 48g; Fiber: 13; Fat: 3g; Protein: 3; Sugar: 28

Peach and Coconut Smoothie

Preparation **Time**: 5 minutes

Servings: 2

Ingredients:

1 cup ice

2 peaches; peeled and chopped

Lemon zest to the taste

1 cup cold coconut milk

1 drop lemon essential oil

Directions:

In your kitchen blender, mix coconut milk with ice and peaches and pulse a few times.

Add lemon zest to the taste and 1 drop lemon essential oil and pulse a few more time. Pour into glasses and serve right away.

Nutrition Values: Calories: 200; Fat: 5g; Fiber: 4g; Carbs: 6g; Protein: 8g

Bacon And Egg Breakfast Sandwich

Preparation **Time**: 20 minutes

Servings: 2

Ingredients:

2 cups bell peppers; chopped

1/2 tbsp. avocado oil

3 eggs

4 bacon slices

Directions:

Heat up a pan with the oil over medium high heat, add bell peppers, stir and cook until they are soft.

Heat up another pan over medium heat, add bacon, stir and cook until it's crispy.

In a bowl; whisk eggs really well and add them to bell peppers.

Cook until eggs are done for about 8 minutes. Divide half of the bacon slices between plates, add eggs, top with bacon slices and serve.

Nutrition Values: Calories: 200; Fat: 4g; Fiber: 3g; Carbs: 6g; Protein: 10g

Lunch/dinner

Korma Curry

Preparation Time: 10 minutes

Cooking time: 25 minutes

Servings: 6

Ingredients:

3-pound chicken breast, skinless, boneless

1 teaspoon garam masala

1 teaspoon curry powder

1 tablespoon apple cider vinegar

½ coconut cream

1 cup organic almond milk

1 teaspoon ground coriander

¾ teaspoon ground cardamom

½ teaspoon ginger powder

¼ teaspoon cayenne pepper

¾ teaspoon ground cinnamon

1 tomato, diced

1 teaspoon avocado oil

½ cup of water

Directions:

Chop the chicken breast and put it in the saucepan.

Add avocado oil and start to cook it over the medium heat.

Sprinkle the chicken with garam masala, curry powder, apple cider vinegar, ground coriander, cardamom, ginger powder, cayenne pepper, ground cinnamon, and diced tomato. Mix up the ingredients carefully. Cook them for 10 minutes.

Add water, coconut cream, and almond milk. Saute the meal for 10 minutes more.

Nutrition Values: calories 411, fat 19.3, fiber 0.9, carbs 6, protein 49.9

Zucchini Bars

Preparation Time: 10 minutes

Cooking time: 15 minutes

Servings: 8

Ingredients:

3 zucchini, grated

½ white onion, diced

2 teaspoons butter

3 eggs, whisked

4 tablespoons coconut flour

1 teaspoon salt

½ teaspoon ground black pepper

5 oz goat cheese, crumbled

4 oz Swiss cheese, shredded

½ cup spinach, chopped

1 teaspoon baking powder

½ teaspoon lemon juice

Directions:

In the mixing bowl, mix up together grated zucchini, diced onion, eggs, coconut flour, salt, ground black pepper, crumbled cheese, chopped spinach, baking powder, and lemon juice.

Add butter and churn the mixture until homogenous.

Line the baking dish with baking paper.

Transfer the zucchini mixture in the baking dish and flatten it.

Preheat the oven to 365F and put the dish inside.

Cook it for 15 minutes. Then chill the meal well.

Cut it into bars.

Nutrition Values: calories 199, fat 1316, fiber 215, carbs 7.1, protein 13.1

Mushroom Soup

Preparation Time: 10 minutes

Cooking time: 25 minutes

Servings: 4

Ingredients:

1 cup of water

1 cup of coconut milk

1 cup white mushrooms, chopped

½ carrot, chopped

¼ white onion, diced

1 tablespoon butter

2 oz turnip, chopped

1 teaspoon dried dill

½ teaspoon ground black pepper

¾ teaspoon smoked paprika

1 oz celery stalk, chopped

Directions:

Pour water and coconut milk in the saucepan. Bring the liquid to boil. Add chopped mushrooms, carrot, and turnip. Close the lid and boil for 10 minutes.

Meanwhile, put butter in the skillet. Add diced onion. Sprinkle it with dill, ground black pepper, and smoked paprika. Roast the onion for 3 minutes.

Add the roasted onion in the soup mixture.

Then add chopped celery stalk. Close the lid.

Cook soup for 10 minutes.

Then ladle it into the serving bowls.

Nutrition Values: calories 181, fat 17.3, fiber 2.5, carbs 6.9, protein 2.4

Stuffed Portobello Mushrooms

Preparation Time: 10 minutes

Cooking time: 10 minutes

Servings: 4

Ingredients:

2 portobello mushrooms

1 cup spinach, chopped, steamed

2 oz artichoke hearts, drained, chopped

1 tablespoon coconut cream

1 tablespoon cream cheese

1 teaspoon minced garlic

1 tablespoon fresh cilantro, chopped

3 oz Cheddar cheese, grated

½ teaspoon ground black pepper

2 tablespoons olive oil

½ teaspoon salt

Directions:

Sprinkle mushrooms with olive oil and place in the tray.

Transfer the tray in the preheated to 360F oven and broil them for 5 minutes.

Meanwhile, blend together artichoke hearts, coconut cream, cream cheese, minced garlic, and chopped cilantro.

Add grated cheese in the mixture and sprinkle with ground black pepper and salt.

Fill the broiled mushrooms with the cheese mixture and cook them for 5 minutes more. Serve the mushrooms only hot.

Nutrition Values: calories 183, fat 16.3, fiber 1.9, carbs 3, protein 7.7

Lettuce Salad

Preparation Time: 10 minutes

Servings: 1

Ingredients:

1 cup Romaine lettuce, roughly chopped

3 oz seitan, chopped

1 tablespoon avocado oil

1 teaspoon sunflower seeds

1 teaspoon lemon juice

1 egg, boiled, peeled

2 oz Cheddar cheese, shredded

Directions:

Place lettuce in the salad bowl. Add chopped seitan and shredded cheese.

Then chop the egg roughly and add in the salad bowl too.

Mix up together lemon juice with the avocado oil.

Sprinkle the salad with the oil mixture and sunflower seeds. Don't stir the salad before serving.

Nutrition Values: calories 663, fat 29.5, fiber 4.7, carbs 3.8, protein 84.2

Onion Soup

Preparation Time: 10 minutes

Cooking time: 25 minutes

Servings: 6

Ingredients:

2 cups white onion, diced

4 tablespoon butter

½ cup white mushrooms, chopped

3 cups of water

1 cup heavy cream

1 teaspoon salt

1 teaspoon chili flakes

1 teaspoon garlic powder

Directions:

Put butter in the saucepan and melt it.

Add diced white onion, chili flakes, and garlic powder. Mix it up and saute for 10 minutes over the medium-low heat.

Then add water, heavy cream, and chopped mushrooms. Close the lid.

Cook the soup for 15 minutes more.

Then blend the soup until you get the creamy texture. Ladle it in the bowls.

Nutrition Values: calories 155, fat 15.1, fiber 0.9, carbs 4.7, protein 1.2

Asparagus Salad

Preparation Time: 10 minutes

Cooking time: 15 minutes

Servings: 3

Ingredients:

10 oz asparagus

1 tablespoon olive oil

½ teaspoon white pepper

4 oz Feta cheese, crumbled

1 cup lettuce, chopped

1 tablespoon canola oil

1 teaspoon apple cider vinegar

1 tomato, diced

Directions:

Preheat the oven to 365F.

Place asparagus in the tray, sprinkle with olive oil and white pepper and transfer in the preheated oven. Cook it for 15 minutes.

Meanwhile, put crumbled Feta in the salad bowl.

Add chopped lettuce and diced tomato.

Sprinkle the ingredients with apple cider vinegar.

Chill the cooked asparagus to the room temperature and add in the salad.

Shake the salad gently before serving.

Nutrition Values: calories 207, fat 17.6, fiber 2.4, carbs 6.8, protein 7.8

Dessert

Keto Cheesecakes

Preparation **Time:** 25 minutes

Servings: 9

Ingredients:

For the cheesecakes:

2 tablespoons butter

1 tablespoon caramel syrup; sugar free

3 tablespoons coffee

8 ounces cream cheese

1/3 cup swerve

3 eggs

For the frosting:

8 ounces mascarpone cheese; soft

3 tablespoons caramel syrup; sugar free

2 tablespoons swerve

3 tablespoons butter

Directions:

In your blender, mix cream cheese with eggs, 2 tablespoons butter, coffee, 1 tablespoon caramel syrup and 1/3 cup swerve and pulse very well.

Spoon this into a cupcakes pan, introduce in the oven at 350 degrees F and bake for 15 minutes

Leave aside to cool down and then keep in the freezer for 3 hours

Meanwhile; in a bowl, mix 3 tablespoons butter with 3 tablespoons caramel syrup, 2 tablespoons swerve and mascarpone cheese and blend well.

Spoon this over cheesecakes and serve them.

Nutrition Values: Calories: 254; Fat : 23; Fiber : 0; Carbs : 1; Protein : 5

Easy Keto Dessert

Preparation **Time:** 40 minutes

Servings: 4

Ingredients:

1/3 cup cocoa powder

1/3 cup erythritol

1 egg

1/4 cup almond flour

1/4 cup walnuts

1/2 teaspoon baking powder

7 tablespoons ghee

1/2 teaspoon vanilla extract

1 tablespoon peanut butter

A pinch of salt

Directions:

Heat up a pan with 6 tablespoons ghee and the erythritol over medium heat; stir and cook for 5 minutes

Transfer this to a bowl, add salt, vanilla extract and cocoa powder and whisk well.

Add egg and stir well again.

Add baking powder, walnuts and almond flour; stir the whole thing really well and pour into a skillet.

In a bowl, mix 1 tablespoon ghee with peanut butter, heat up in your microwave for a few seconds and stir well.

Drizzle this over brownies mix in the skillet, introduce in the oven at 350 degrees F and bake for 30 minutes

Leave brownies to cool down, cut and serve

Nutrition Values: Calories: 223; Fat : 32; Fiber : 1; Carbs : 3; Protein : 6

Keto Brownies

Preparation **Time:** 30 minutes

Servings: 12

Ingredients:

6 ounces coconut oil; melted

4 ounces cream cheese

5 tablespoons swerve

6 eggs

2 teaspoons vanilla

3 ounces cocoa powder

1/2 teaspoon baking powder

Directions:

In a blender, mix eggs with coconut oil, cocoa powder, baking powder, vanilla, cream cheese and swerve and stir using a mixer.

Pour this into a lined baking dish, introduce in the oven at 350 degrees F and bake for 20 minutes

Slice into rectangle pieces when their cold and serve

Nutrition Values: Calories: 178; Fat: 14; Fiber: 2; Carbs: 3; Protein : 5

Raspberry and Coconut

Preparation **Time:** 15 minutes

Servings: 12

Ingredients:

1/4 cup swerve

1/2 cup coconut oil

1/2 cup raspberries; dried

1/2 cup coconut; shredded

1/2 cup coconut butter

Directions:

In your food processor, blend dried berries very well.

Heat up a pan with the butter over medium heat.

Add oil, coconut and swerve; stir and cook for 5 minutes

Pour half of this into a lined baking pan and spread well.

Add raspberry powder and also spread.

Top with the rest of the butter mix, spread and keep in the fridge for a while Cut into pieces and serve

Nutrition Values: Calories: 234; Fat : 22; Fiber : 2; Carbs : 4; Protein : 2

Chocolate Pudding Delight

Preparation **Time:** 52 minutes

Servings: 2

Ingredients:

1/2 teaspoon stevia powder

2 tablespoons cocoa powder

2 tablespoons water

1 tablespoon gelatin

1 cup coconut milk

2 tablespoons maple syrup

Directions:

Heat up a pan with the coconut milk over medium heat; add stevia and cocoa powder and stir well.

In a bowl, mix gelatin with water; stir well and add to the pan.

Stir well, add maple syrup, whisk again, divide into ramekins and keep in the fridge for 45 minutes Serve cold.

Nutrition Values: Calories: 140; Fat : 2; Fiber : 2; Carbs : 4; Protein : 4

Special Keto Pudding

Preparation Time: 4 hours 13 minutes

Servings: 2

Ingredients:

1 cup coconut milk

4 teaspoons gelatin

1/4 teaspoon ginger; ground

1/4 teaspoon liquid stevia

A pinch of nutmeg; ground

A pinch of cardamom; ground

Directions:

In a bowl, mix 1/4 cup milk with gelatin and stir well.

Put the rest of the coconut milk in a pot and heat up over medium heat.

Add gelatin mix; stir, take off heat; leave aside to cool down and then keep in the fridge for 4 hours

Transfer this to a food processor, add stevia, cardamom, nutmeg and ginger and blend for a couple of minutes

Divide into dessert cups and serve cold.

Nutrition Values: Calories: 150; Fat : 1; Fiber : 0; Carbs : 2; Protein : 6

Peanut Butter Fudge

Preparation **Time:** 2 hours 12 minutes

Servings: 12

Ingredients:

1 cup peanut butter; unsweetened

1 cup coconut oil

1/4 cup almond milk

2 teaspoons vanilla stevia

A pinch of salt

For the topping:

2 tablespoons swerve

1/4 cup cocoa powder

2 tablespoons melted coconut oil

Directions:

In a heat proof bowl, mix peanut butter with 1 cup coconut oil; stir and heat up in your microwave until it melts

Add a pinch of salt, almond milk and stevia; stir well everything and pour into a lined loaf pan.

Keep in the fridge for 2 hours and then slice it.

In a bowl, mix 2 tablespoons melted coconut with cocoa powder and swerve and stir very well.

Drizzle the sauce over your peanut butter fudge and serve

Nutrition Values: Calories: 265; Fat : 23; Fiber : 2; Carbs : 4; Protein : 6

Conclusion

If you are over 50's, then you know how difficult it is to maintain health and shed that extra weight. Whether you are going through menopause, have more time to eat and socialize, dropping weight after 50s is not a piece of cake.

If nothing else is working, give the ketogenic diet a try. The fact is that millions of people have successfully implemented a high-fat keto diet as a way to lose weight. It's highly effective because it turns your body into a natural fat burner, without leaving you hungry, craving for sugary foods, or suffering from health effects due to too few calories.

With the keto diet, imagine a life with less and less belly fat.

Imagine eating as much as you want, every single day, and still watch your waist and stomach shrink.

And, imagine yourself active and energetic as you were in your 20's and 30's.

Made in the USA
Columbia, SC
07 January 2020